CW00506703

LOW FAT AIR FRYER

FRYER

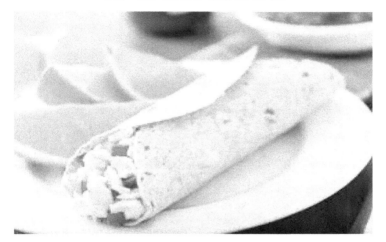

BREAKFAST

MEAL PREP

Celine Montero

Welcome!

"Low Fat Air Fryer Meal Prep" is a series I created to walk you through delicious recipes selected by myself.

As you may already know, the air fryer is a fantastic tool anybody can use to quickly prepare our meals, through a healthy cooking method.

The fact is that's the latest hottest kitchen appliance .

BENEFITS OF THE AIR FRYER

- ## *Less Cooking Time*

It cooks your food using the fan to circulate the hot air on all parts of your food. Thanks to the design, it cooks faster than a regular oven. You are able to cook your meal in 15mins, while it takes much more to do in in an oven.

• *Energy Efficient*

When there's a heatwave you will have the air fryer cook without influencing your home temperature. most people prefer to work with gadgets that show to be environmentally friendly - This is one such gadget. Hence most people prefer the air fryer rather than a regular oven.

• *Super Easy To Clean*

For those people with problems of cleaning, do not worry at all because you won't have to spend much time cleaning with this gadget.

You can place the parts directly in your dishwasher.

• *Super Easy To Use*

Most of the air fryers have only 2 buttons to control the entire appliance. The only two things you need to do are setting the temperature and time, then let the food cook after you shaked it a few times.

• *It Is Versatile*

With just the air fryer, you can deep fry the food, stir fry, reheat, broil, bake or roast it. You cannot have in your kitchen tools able do only one thing or cook just one kind of food.

The recipes this series of books contains are selected and divided by categories in 8 cookbooks, to made you enjoy as best this (in my opinion) revolutionary way to cook foods.

I hope you will enjoy and find all these recipes interesting and helpful to set up your daily meal plan.

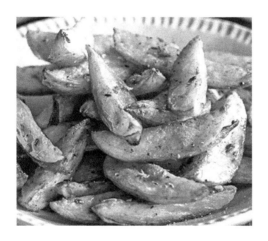

Celine Montero

5

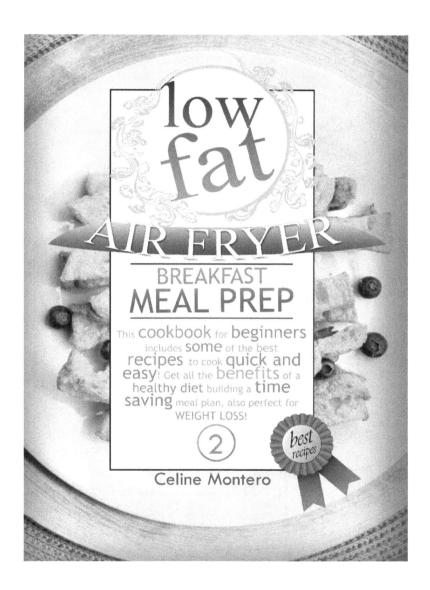

low fat

AIR FRYER

BREAKFAST
MEAL PREP

This cookbook for beginners includes some of the best recipes to cook quick and easy! Get all the benefits of a healthy diet building a time saving meal plan, also perfect for WEIGHT LOSS!

(2)

best recipes

Celine Montero

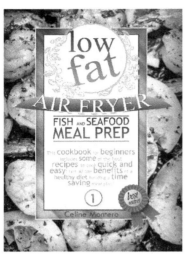

LOW FAT AIR FRYER
FISH AND SEAFOOD MEAL PREP

This cookbook for beginners includes some of the best recipes to cook quick and easy! Get all the benefits of a healthy diet building a time saving meal plan!

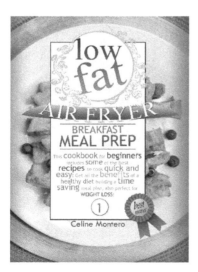

LOW FAT AIR FRYER
BREAKFAST MEAL PREP

This cookbook for beginners includes some of the best recipes to cook quick and easy! Get all the benefits of a healthy diet building a time saving meal plan, also perfect for weight loss!

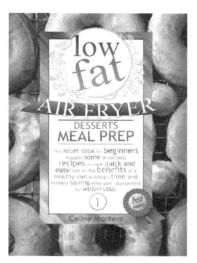

LOW FAT AIR FRYER
DESSERTS MEAL PREP

This recipe book for beginners includes some of the best recipes to cook quick and easy! Get all the benefits of a healthy diet building a time and money saving meal plan, also perfect for weight loss!

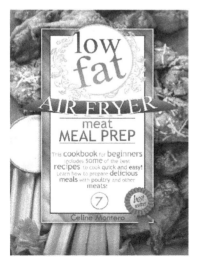

LOW FAT AIR FRYER
MEAT MEAL PREP

This cookbook for beginners includes some of the best recipes to cook quick and easy! Learn how to prepare delicious meals with poultry and other meats!

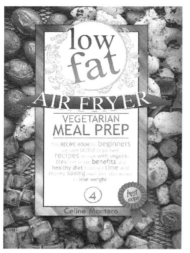

LOW FAT AIR FRYER
VEGETARIAN MEAL PREP

This recipe book for beginners includes some of the best recipes to cook with vegetables! Get all the benefits of a healthy diet building a time and money saving meal plan, also perfect to lose weight!

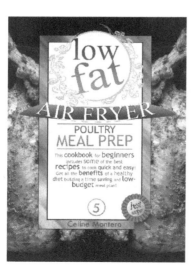

LOW FAT AIR FRYER
POULTRY MEAL PREP

This cookbook for beginners includes some of the best recipes to cook quick and easy! Get all the benefits of a healthy diet building a time saving and low-budget meal plan!

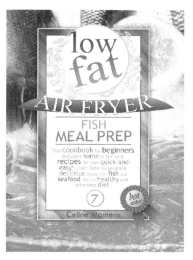

LOW FAT AIR FRYER
POULTRY MEAL PREP

This cookbook for beginners includes some of the best recipes to cook quick-and-easy! Learn how to prepare delicious meals with fish and seafood,
for a healthy and effortless diet!

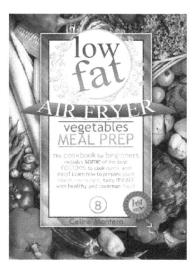

LOW FAT AIR FRYER
VEGETABLES MEAL PREP

This cookbook for beginners includes some of the best recipes to cook quick-and-easy! Learn how to prepare plant-based, low-budget and tasty meals, with healthy and common food, ideal for weight loss!

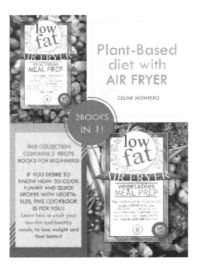

PLANT-BASED DIET WITH AIR FRYER

This collection contains 2 recipe books for beginners! If you desire to know how to cook yummy and quick recipes with vegetables, this cookbook is for you! Learn how to cook your low-fat and healthy meals, to lose weight and feel better!

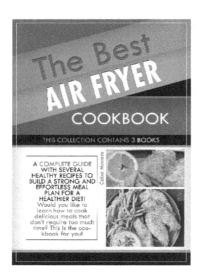

THE BEST AIR FRYER COOKBOOK

THIS COLLECTION CONTAINS 3 BOOKS: a complete guide with several healthy recipes to build a strong and effortless meal plan for a healthier diet! Would you like to learn how to cook delicious meals that don't require too much time? This is the cookbook for you!

Table of Contents

14

START YOUR DAY
WITH
THE RIGHT FOOT

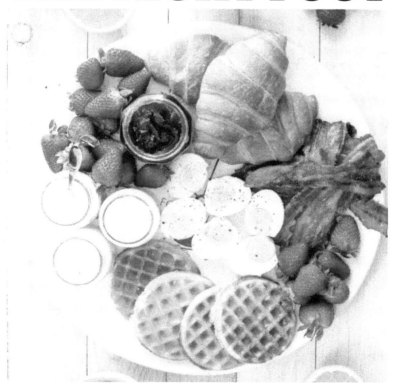

Coconut & Oat Cookies

Prep + Cook Time: 30 minutes 4 Servings

Ingredients

- ¾ cup flour
- 4 tbsp sugar
- ½ cup oats 1 egg ¼ cup coconut flakes
- Filling:
- 1 tbsp white chocolate, melted
- 4 tbsp butter ½ cup powdered sugar
- 1 tsp vanilla extract

Directions

In a bowl, beat egg, sugar, oats, and coconut flakes with an electric mixer. Fold in the flour. Drop spoonfuls of the

18

batter onto a greased baking sheet and cook in the air fryer at 350 F for 18 minutes on Bake. Let cool to firm up and resemble cookies. Cook in batches if needed. Meanwhile, prepare the filling by beating all ingredients together. Spread the filling on half of the cookies. Top with the other halves to make cookie sandwiches.

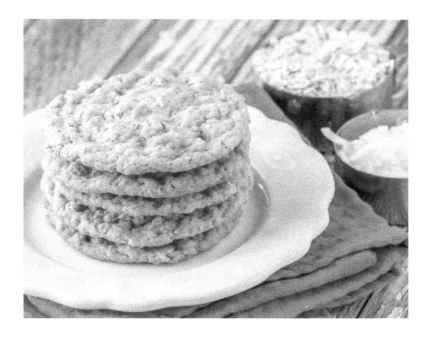

Paprika Rarebit

Prep + Cook Time: 15 minutes 2 Servings

Ingredients

- 4 slices bread, toasted
- 1 tsp smoked paprika
- 2 eggs, beaten
- 1 tsp dijon mustard
- 4 ½ oz cheddar cheese, grated
- Salt and black pepper to taste

Directions

In a bowl, combine the eggs, mustard, cheddar cheese, and paprika. Season with salt and pepper. Spread the mixture on the toasts. AirFry the slices in the preheated air fryer for 10 minutes at 360 F.

Quick Feta Triangles

Prep + Cook Time: 30 minutes 3 Servings

Ingredients

- 1 cup feta cheese
- 1 onion, chopped
- 2 tbsp parsley, chopped
- 1 egg yolk
- 2 tbsp olive oil
- 3 sheets filo pastry

Directions Cut each of the filo sheets into 3 equal-sized strips. Brush the strips with some olive oil. In a bowl, mix onion, feta, egg yolk, and parsley. Divide the mixture between the strips and fold each diagonally to make triangles. Arrange them on a greased baking pan and brush the tops with the remaining olive oil. Place in the fryer and Bake for 8 minutes at 360 F. Serve warm.

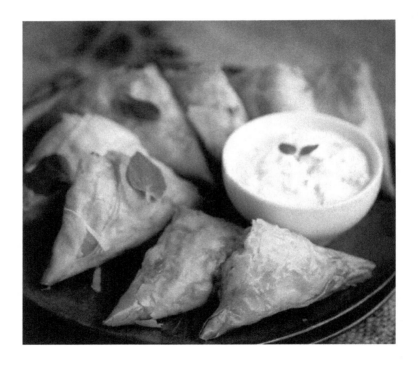

Turkey Sausage

Preparation Time: 10 minutes Cooking Time: 10 minutes Serve: 8

Ingredients:

- 2 lbs ground turkey

- 1 tsp dried thyme

- 1 tsp paprika

- 2 tsp garlic powder

- 2 tsp dry sage

- 2 tsp fennel seeds

- 1 tsp sea salt

Directions:

Add ground meat and remaining ingredients into the mixing bowl and mix until well combined. Take 2-3 tablespoon of meat mixture and flatten into patties. Place the cooking tray in the air fryer basket. Select Air Fry mode. Set time to 10 minutes and temperature 370 F then press START. The air fryer display will prompt you to ADD FOOD once the temperature is reached then place sausage patties in the air fryer basket. Serve and enjoy. Nutritional Value (Amount per Serving

Savory Breakfast Casserole

Preparation Time: 10 minutes Cooking Time: 45 minutes Serve: 8

Ingredients:

- 12 eggs

- 1 tbsp hot sauce

- 3/4 cup heavy whipping cream

- 2 cups cheddar cheese, shredded

- 12 oz breakfast sausage

- Pepper Salt

Directions:

Heat large pan over medium-high heat. Add sausage in a pan and cook for 5-7 minutes or until meat is no longer pink. Add cooked sausage in a 9*13-inch baking dish. In a large bowl, whisk eggs with hot sauce, cream, cheese, pepper, and salt. Pour egg mixture over sausage in baking dish. Cover dish with foil. Select Bake mode. Set time to 40 minutes and temperature 350 F then press START. The air fryer display will prompt you to ADD FOOD once the temperature is reached then place the baking dish in the air fryer basket. Serve and enjoy.

Zucchini Spinach Egg Casserole

Preparation Time: 10 minutes Cooking Time: 30 minutes Serve: 8

Ingredients:

- 10 eggs

- 1/4 cup goat cheese, crumbled

- 4 cherry tomatoes, cut in half

- 1/3 cup cheddar cheese, grated

- 1/3 cup ham, chopped

- 1 small zucchini, sliced

- 1/2 cup spinach

- 2/3 cup heavy cream

- Pepper Salt

Directions:

In a bowl, whisk eggs with cream, pepper, and salt. Stir in cheddar cheese, ham, zucchini, and spinach. Pour egg mixture into the greased baking dish. Top with goat cheese and cherry tomatoes. Cover dish with foil. Select Bake mode. Set time to 30 minutes and temperature 350 F then press START. The air fryer display will prompt you to ADD FOOD once the temperature is reached then place the baking dish in the air fryer basket. Serve and enjoy.

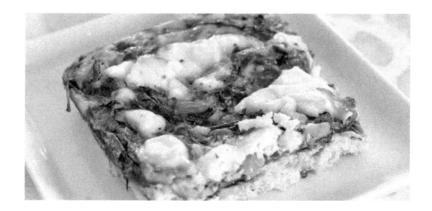

Ham Cheese Casserole

Preparation Time: 10 minutes Cooking Time: 35 minutes Serve: 12

Ingredients:

- 12 eggs

- 1/2 cup cheddar cheese, shredded

- 4 oz cream cheese, cubed

- 2 cups ham, diced

- 1 cup heavy cream

- 1/4 tsp pepper

- 1/4 tsp salt

Directions:

In a large bowl, whisk eggs with cream, pepper, and salt. Stir in cheddar cheese, cream cheese, and ham. Pour egg mixture into the greased 9*13-inch baking dish. Cover dish with foil. Select Bake mode. Set time to 35 minutes and temperature 350 F then press START. The air fryer display will prompt you to ADD FOOD once the temperature is reached then place the baking dish in the air fryer basket. Serve and enjoy.

Crustless Cheese Egg Quiche

Preparation Time: 10 minutes Cooking Time: 45 minutes Serve: 6

Ingredients:

- 12 eggs

- 12 tbsp butter, melted

- 4 oz cream cheese, softened

- 8 oz cheddar cheese, grated

- Pepper Salt

Directions:

In a bowl, whisk eggs with butter, cream cheese, half cheddar cheese, pepper, and salt. Pour egg mixture into the greased 9.5-inch pie pan. Sprinkle remaining cheese on top. Cover dish with foil. Select Bake mode. Set time to 45 minutes and temperature 325 F then press START. The air fryer display will prompt you to ADD FOOD once the temperature is reached then place the pie pan in the air fryer basket. Serve and enjoy.

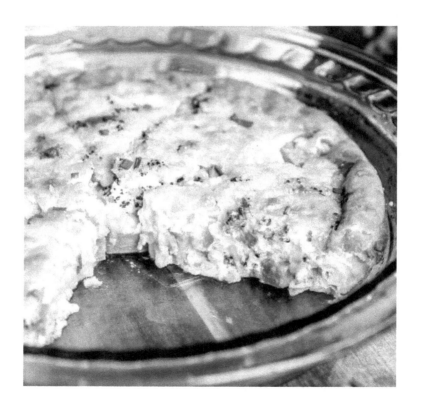

Veggie Egg Casserole

Preparation Time: 10 minutes Cooking Time: 30 minutes Serve: 10

Ingredients:

- 12 eggs, lightly beaten

- 1 cup cheddar cheese, shredded

- 2 bell pepper, diced

- 1 tsp garlic, minced

- 1 cup onion, chopped

- 5 bacon slices, cooked and chopped

- 1 tbsp olive oil

- 1/4 tsp pepper

- 1/2 tsp sea salt

Directions:

Heat oil in a pan over medium heat. Add garlic and onion in a pan and sauté until onion is softened. In a bowl, whisk eggs with pepper and salt. Stir in cheddar cheese, bell pepper, bacon, garlic, and onion. Pour egg mixture into the greased 9*13-inch baking dish. Cover dish with foil. Select Bake mode. Set time to 30 minutes and temperature 350 F then press START. The air fryer display will prompt you to ADD FOOD once the temperature is reached then place the baking dish in the air fryer basket. Serve and enjoy.

Cauliflower Muffins

Preparation Time: 10 minutes Cooking Time: 25 minutes Serve: 12

Ingredients:

- 5 eggs

- 1 cup cheddar cheese, shredded

- 1/2 tsp garlic powder

- 1/2 cup onion, chopped

- 1/2 cup baby spinach

- 6 oz ham, diced

- 3 cups cauliflower rice, squeeze out excess liquid

- Pepper Salt

Directions:

In a bowl, whisk eggs with cheese, garlic powder, pepper, and salt. Stir in onion, spinach, ham, and cauliflower rice. Pour egg mixture into the silicone muffin molds. Select Bake mode. Set time to 25 minutes and temperature 375 F then press START. The air fryer display will prompt you to ADD FOOD once the temperature is reached then place muffin molds in the air fryer basket. Serve and enjoy.

Delicious Zucchini Frittata

Preparation Time: 10 minutes Cooking Time: 30 minutes Serve: 4

Ingredients:

- 8 eggs

- 1 tbsp parsley, chopped

- 3 tbsp parmesan cheese, grated

- 2 small zucchinis, grated

- 1/2 cup pancetta, chopped

- 2 tbsp olive oil

- Pepper Salt

Directions:

Heat oil in a pan over medium heat. Add zucchini and pancetta into the pan and sauté for 8-10 minutes. In a bowl, whisk eggs with parsley, cheese, pepper, and salt. Stir in sauteed zucchini and pancetta. Pour egg mixture into the greased 8-inch baking dish. Select Bake mode. Set time to 20 minutes and temperature 350 F then press START. The air fryer display will prompt you to ADD FOOD once the temperature is reached then place the baking dish in the air fryer basket. Serve and enjoy.

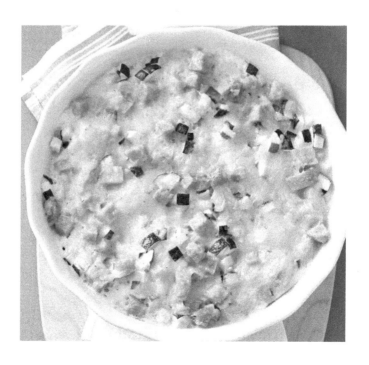

Cheesy Zucchini Quiche

Preparation Time: 10 minutes Cooking Time: 60 minutes Serve: 8

Ingredients:

- 6 eggs

- 2 medium zucchinis, shredded & Squeeze out excess liquid

- 2 tbsp fresh parsley, chopped

- 1/2 cup olive oil

- 1 cup cheddar cheese, shredded

- 1 cup almond flour

- 1/2 tsp dried basil

- 2 garlic cloves, minced

- 1 tbsp dry onion, minced

- 2 tbsp parmesan cheese, grated

- 1/2 tsp salt

Directions:

Add all ingredients into the large bowl and mix until well combined. Pour mixture into the greased 9-inch pie dish. Cover pie dish with foil. Select Bake mode. Set time to 60 minutes and temperature 350 F then press START. The air fryer display will prompt you to ADD FOOD once the temperature is reached then place the pie dish in the air fryer basket. Slice and serve.

Tomato Kale Egg Muffins

Preparation Time: 10 minutes Cooking Time: 25 minutes Serve: 6

Ingredients:

- 5 eggs

- 3 tomatoes, chopped

- 2/3 cup unsweetened almond milk

- 1 green onion, chopped

- 1/2 cup kale, shredded

- 1/8 tsp pepper

- 1/4 tsp salt

Directions:

In a bowl, whisk eggs with milk, pepper, and salt. Stir in tomatoes, kale, and onion. Pour egg mixture into the silicone muffin molds. Select Bake mode. Set time to 25 minutes and temperature 350 F then press START. The air fryer display will prompt you to ADD FOOD once the temperature is reached then place muffin molds in the air fryer basket. Serve and enjoy.

Healthy Breakfast Donuts

Preparation Time: 10 minutes Cooking Time: 20 minutes Serve: 6

Ingredients:

- 4 eggs

- 1/2 tsp instant coffee

- 1/3 cup unsweetened almond milk

- 1 tbsp liquid stevia

- 3 tbsp cocoa powder

- 1/4 cup butter, melted

- 1/3 cup coconut flour

- 1/2 tsp baking soda

- 1/2 tsp baking powder

Directions:

Add all ingredients into the large bowl and mix until well combined. Pour batter into the silicone donut molds. Select Bake mode. Set time to 20 minutes and temperature 350 F then press START. The air fryer display will prompt you to ADD FOOD once the temperature is reached then place donut molds in the air fryer basket. Serve and enjoy.

Simple & Easy Breakfast Quiche

Preparation Time: 10 minutes Cooking Time: 45 minutes Serve: 6

Ingredients:

- 6 eggs

- 1 cup unsweetened almond milk

- 1 cup tomatoes, chopped

- 1 cup cheddar cheese, grated

- 1 tsp garlic powder

- Pepper Salt

Directions:

In a bowl, whisk eggs with cheese, milk, garlic powder, pepper, and salt. Stir in tomatoes. Pour egg mixture into the greased pie dish. Cover dish with foil. Select Bake mode. Set time to 45 minutes and temperature 350 F then press START. The air fryer display will prompt you to ADD FOOD once the temperature is reached then place the pie dish in the air fryer basket. Serve and enjoy.

Parmesan Zucchini Frittata

Preparation Time: 10 minutes Cooking Time: 30 minutes Serve: 4

Ingredients:

- 8 eggs

- 2 zucchinis, chopped and cooked

- 1 tbsp fresh parsley, chopped

- 3 tbsp parmesan cheese, grated

- 1 tsp garlic powder

- Pepper Salt

Directions:

In a large bowl, whisk eggs with garlic powder, pepper, and salt. Stir in parsley, cheese, and zucchini. Pour egg mixture into the greased baking dish. Cover dish with foil. Select Bake mode. Set time to 30 minutes and temperature 350 F then press START. The air fryer display will prompt you to ADD FOOD once the temperature is reached then place the baking dish in the air fryer basket. Serve and enjoy

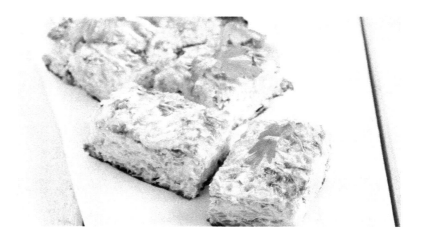

Bake Cheese Omelet

Preparation Time: 10 minutes Cooking Time: 25 minutes Serve: 6

Ingredients:

- 8 eggs

- 1/4 cup cheddar cheese, shredded

- 2 tbsp green onions, chopped

- 1/4 tsp garlic powder

- 1/2 cup unsweetened almond milk

- 1/2 cup half and half

- Pepper Salt

Directions:

In a bowl, whisk eggs with milk, half and half, garlic powder, pepper, and salt. Stir in green onion and cheese. Pour egg mixture into the greased 8-inch baking dish. Cover dish with foil. Select Bake mode. Set time to 25 minutes and temperature 350 F then press START. The air fryer display will prompt you to ADD FOOD once the temperature is reached then place the baking dish in the air fryer basket. Serve and enjoy.

Sun-dried Tomatoes Egg Cups

Preparation Time: 10 minutes Cooking Time: 20 minutes Serve: 12

Ingredients:

- 6 eggs

- 1 1/2 tbsp basil, chopped

- 2 tsp olive oil

- 1/2 cup feta cheese, crumbled

- 4 cherry tomatoes, chopped

- 4 sun-dried tomatoes, chopped

- Pepper Salt

Directions:

In a bowl, whisk eggs with pepper and salt. Add remaining ingredients and stir well. Pour egg mixture into the silicone muffin molds. Select Bake mode. Set time to 20 minutes and temperature 400 F then press START. The air fryer display will prompt you to ADD FOOD once the temperature is reached then place muffin molds in the air fryer basket. Serve and enjoy.

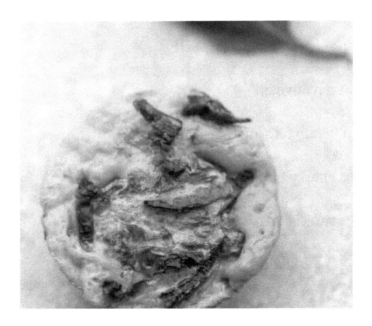

Mushroom Kale Egg Cups

Preparation Time: 10 minutes Cooking Time: 15 minutes Serve: 8

Ingredients:

- 6 eggs

- 1 cup mushrooms, diced

- 1 cup kale, chopped

- 1 tsp olive oil

- 2 tbsp onion, minced

- 1/2 cup Swiss cheese, shredded

- Pepper Salt

Directions:

Heat oil in a pan over medium-high heat. Add mushrooms and sauté for 2-3 minutes. Add onion and kale and sauté for 2 minutes. Remove pan from heat. In a bowl, whisk eggs with pepper and salt. Stir in sautéed mushroom kale mixture and shredded cheese. Pour egg mixture into the silicone muffin molds. Select Bake mode. Set time to 15 minutes and temperature 350 F then press START. The air fryer display will prompt you to ADD FOOD once the temperature is reached then place muffin molds in the air fryer basket. Serve and enjoy.

Sun-dried Tomatoes Kale Egg Cups

Preparation Time: 10 minutes Cooking Time: 35 minutes Serve: 12

Ingredients:

- 10 eggs

- 1/4 cup sun-dried tomatoes, chopped

- 1 cup unsweetened coconut milk

- 1/4 cup sausage, sliced

- 1/4 cup kale, chopped

- Pepper Salt

Directions:

In a large bowl, add all ingredients and whisk until well combined. Pour egg mixture into the silicone muffin molds. Select Bake mode. Set time to 35 minutes and temperature 350 F then press START. The air fryer display will prompt you to ADD FOOD once the temperature is reached then place muffin molds in the air fryer basket. Serve and enjoy.

Roasted Pepper Egg Cups

Preparation Time: 10 minutes Cooking Time: 20 minutes Serve: 12

Ingredients:

- 8 eggs

- 1 cup roasted red peppers, chopped

- 1/4 cup unsweetened almond milk

- 1 cup spinach, chopped

- 1/2 tsp salt

Directions:

In a bowl, whisk eggs with coconut milk and salt. Add spinach, green onion, and red peppers to the egg mixture and stir to combine. Pour egg mixture into the silicone muffin molds. Select Bake mode. Set time to 20 minutes and temperature 350 F then press START. The air fryer display will prompt you to ADD FOOD once the temperature is reached then place muffin molds in the air fryer basket. Serve and enjoy.

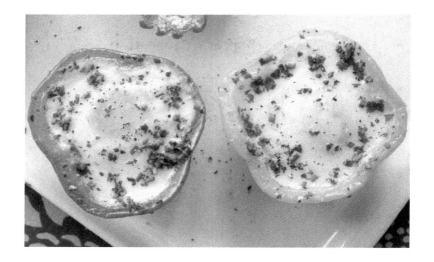

Spinach Bacon Egg Bake

Preparation Time: 10 minutes Cooking Time: 45 minutes Serve: 6

Ingredients:

- 10 eggs

- 3 cups baby spinach, chopped

- 1 tbsp olive oil

- 10 bacon sliced, cooked and crumbled

- 2 large tomatoes, sliced

- 1/2 tsp salt

Directions:

Heat oil in a pan over medium heat. Add spinach and cook until spinach wilted. In a mixing bowl, whisk eggs with salt. Stir in spinach. Pour egg mixture into the greased 9-inch baking dish. Cover dish with foil. Select Bake mode. Set time to 45 minutes and temperature 350 F then press START. The air fryer display will prompt you to ADD FOOD once the temperature is reached then place the baking dish in the air fryer basket. Serve and enjoy.

Egg Casserole

Preparation Time: 10 minutes Cooking Time: 30 minutes Serve: 2

Ingredients:

- 5 eggs

- 2 tbsp heavy cream

- 3 tbsp tomato sauce

- 2 tbsp parmesan cheese, grated

Directions:

In a bowl, whisk eggs with cream. Stir in cheese and tomato sauce. Pour egg mixture into the greased baking dish. Cover dish with foil. Select Bake mode. Set time to 30 minutes and temperature 350 F then press START. The air fryer display will prompt you to ADD FOOD once the temperature is reached then place the baking dish in the air fryer basket. Serve and enjoy.

Spinach Egg Bake

Preparation Time: 10 minutes Cooking Time: 35 minutes Serve: 6

Ingredients:

- 8 eggs, beaten

- 1 1/2 cups mozzarella

- 1 tsp olive oil

- 5 oz fresh spinach

- 1 tsp spike seasoning

- 1/3 cup green onion, sliced

- Pepper Salt

Directions:

Heat oil in a large pan over medium heat. Add spinach and cook until wilted. Transfer cooked spinach into the casserole dish and spread well. Spread onion and cheese on top. In a bowl, whisk together eggs, pepper, spike seasoning, and salt. Pour egg mixture over spinach mixture. Cover dish with foil. Select Bake mode. Set time to 35 minutes and temperature 375 F then press START. The air fryer display will prompt you to ADD FOOD once the temperature is reached then place a casserole dish in the air fryer basket. Slice and serve.

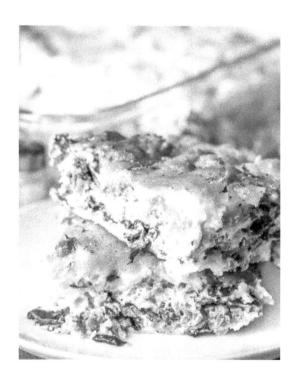

Spinach Pepper Breakfast Egg Cups

Preparation Time: 10 minutes Cooking Time: 20 minutes Serve: 12

Ingredients:

- 9 eggs

- 1 cup bell peppers, chopped

- 1/2 cup onion, sliced

- 1 tbsp olive oil

- 8 oz ground sausage

- 1/4 cup unsweetened almond milk

- 1/2 tsp oregano

- 1 1/2 cups spinach

- Pepper Salt

Directions:

Add ground sausage in a pan and sauté over medium heat until browned. Add olive oil, oregano, bell pepper, and onion and sauté until onion is translucent. Add spinach and cook until spinach is wilted. Remove pan from heat and set aside. In a bowl, whisk eggs, milk, pepper, and salt. Add sausage and vegetable mixture into the egg mixture and mix well. Pour egg mixture into the silicone muffin molds. Select Bake mode. Set time to 20 minutes and temperature 350 F then press START.The air fryer display will prompt you to ADD FOOD once the temperature is reached then place muffin molds in the air fryer basket. Serve and enjoy.

Cheddar Cheese Ham Quiche

Preparation Time: 10 minutes Cooking Time: 40 minutes Serve: 6

Ingredients:

- 8 eggs

- 1 cup zucchini, shredded and squeezed

- 1 cup ham, cooked and diced

- 1/2 tsp dry mustard

- 1/2 cup heavy cream

- 1 cup cheddar cheese, shredded

- Pepper Salt

Directions:

Add ham, cheddar cheese, and zucchini in a 9-inch pie dish. In a bowl, whisk together eggs, heavy cream, and seasoning. Pour egg mixture over ham mixture. Cover dish with foil. Select Bake mode. Set time to 40 minutes and temperature 375 F then press START. The air fryer display will prompt you to ADD FOOD once the temperature is reached then add food in the air fryer basket. Serve and enjoy.

Coconut Jalapeno Muffins

Preparation Time: 10 minutes Cooking Time: 20 minutes Serve: 8

Ingredients:

- 5 eggs

- 3 tbsp jalapenos, sliced

- 3 tbsp erythritol

- 2/3 cup coconut flour

- 1/4 cup unsweetened coconut milk

- 1/3 cup coconut oil, melted

- 2 tsp baking powder

- 3/4 tsp sea salt

Directions:

In a large bowl, stir together coconut flour, baking powder, sweetener, and sea salt. Stir in eggs, jalapenos, milk, and coconut oil until well combined. Pour batter into the silicone muffin molds. Select Bake mode. Set time to 20 minutes and temperature 350 F then press START. The air fryer display will prompt you to ADD FOOD once the temperature is reached then place muffin molds in the air fryer basket. Serve and enjoy.

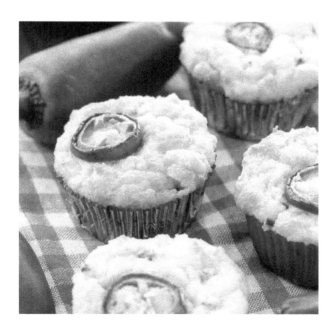

Breakfast Vegetable Quiche

Preparation Time: 10 minutes Cooking Time: 40 minutes Serve: 6

Ingredients:

- 8 egg whites

- 1 cup gruyere cheese, shredded

- 1/4 cup onion, diced

- 2 cups spinach, steamed & squeeze out excess liquid

- 4 pieces roasted red peppers, sliced

- 1/2 cup cherry tomatoes, halved

- 1 garlic cloves, minced

- 1/2 cup unsweetened coconut milk

- Pepper Salt

Directions:

Spray pan with cooking spray and heat over medium-high heat. Add garlic and onion and sauté until softened. In a bowl, whisk egg whites, cheese, and milk. Add sautéed onion and garlic into the egg mixture and stir well. Layer tomatoes, roasted peppers, and spinach in a greased baking dish. Pour egg mixture over the vegetables. Cover dish with foil. Select Bake mode. Set time to 40 minutes and temperature 350 F then press START. The air fryer display will prompt you to ADD FOOD once the temperature is reached then place the baking dish in the air fryer basket. Serve and enjoy.

Mediterranean Avocado Toast

Prep + Cook Time: 7 minutes 2 Serving

Ingredients

- 2 slices thick whole grain bread

- 4 thin tomato slices

- 1 ripe avocado, pitted, peeled, and sliced

- 1 tbsp olive oil

- 1 tbsp pinch of salt

- ½ tsp chili flakes

Directions

Preheat air fryer to 370 F. Arrange the bread slices on the fryer and toast on Bake mode. Add the avocado to a bowl and mash it up with a fork until smooth. Season with salt. When the toasted bread is ready, remove it to a plate. Drizzle with olive oil and arrange the thin tomato slices on top. Spread the avocado mash on top. Sprinkle the toasts with chili flakes and serve

Bacon & Egg Sandwich

Prep + Cook Time: 10 minutes 1 Serving

Ingredients

- 1 egg, fried

- 1 slice English bacon

- Salt and black pepper to taste

- 2 bread slices

- ½ tbsp butter, softened

Directions

Preheat air fryer to 400 F. Spread butter on one side of the bread slices. Add the fried egg on top and season with salt and black pepper. Top with bacon and cover with the other slice of bread. Place in the fryer's cooking basket and AirFry for 4-6 minutes. Serve warm.

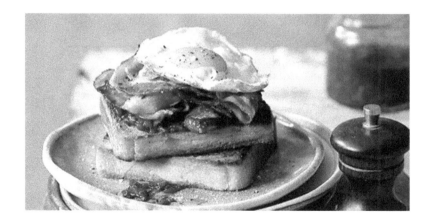

Grilled Apple & Brie Sandwich

Prep + Cook Time: 10 minutes 1 Serving

Ingredients

- 2 bread slices

- ½ apple, thinly sliced

- 2 tsp butter

- 2 oz brie cheese, thinly sliced

Directions

Spread butter on the outside of the bread slices and top with apple slices. Place brie slices on top of the apple and cover with the other slice of bread. Bake in the fryer for 5 minutes at 350 F. When ready, remove and cut diagonally to serve.

Air Fried Sourdough Sandwiches

Prep + Cook Time: 20 minutes 2 Servings

Ingredients

- 4 slices sourdough bread

- 2 tbsp mayonnaise

- 2 slices ham

- 2 lettuce leaves

- 1 tomato, sliced

- 2 slices mozzarella chees

Directions

Preheat air fryer to 350 F. On a clean working board, lay the bread slices and spread them with mayonnaise. Top 2 of the slices with ham, lettuce leaves, tomato slices, and mozzarella. Cover with the remaining bread slices to form two sandwiches. AirFry for 12 minutes, flipping once. Serve hot.

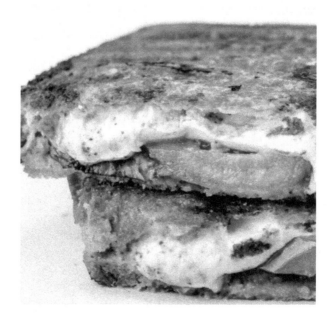

Sausage & Egg Casserole

Prep + Cook Time: 20 minutes 6 Servings

Ingredients

- 1 lb ground sausages

- 6 eggs

- 1 red pepper, diced

- 1 green pepper, diced

- 1 yellow pepper, diced

- 1 sweet onion, diced

- 1 cup cheddar cheese, shredded

- Salt and black pepper to taste

- 2 tbsp fresh parsley, chopped

Directions

Place a skillet over medium heat on a stovetop. Add the sausages and cook until brown, turning occasionally, about 5 minutes. Once done, drain any excess fat derived from cooking and set aside. Arrange the sausages on the bottom of a greased casserole dish that fits in your air fryer. Top with onion, red pepper, green pepper, and yellow pepper. Sprinkle the cheese on top. In a bowl, beat the eggs with salt and pepper. Pour the mixture over the cheese. Place the casserole dish in the air fryer basket and bake at 360 F for 15 minutes. Serve warm garnished with fresh parsley.

Cheese & Ham Breakfast Egg Cups

Prep + Cook Time: 20 minutes 6 Servings

Ingredients

- 4 eggs, beaten

- 1 tbsp olive oil

- ½ cup Colby cheese, shredded

- 2 ¼ cups frozen hash browns, thawed

- 1 cup smoked ham, chopped

- ½ tsp Cajun seasoning

Directions

Preheat air fryer to 360 F. Gather 12 silicone muffin cups and coat with olive oil. Whisk the eggs, hash browns, smoked ham, Colby cheese, and Cajun seasoning in a medium bowl and add a heaping spoonful into each muffin cup. Put the muffin cups in the fryer basket and AirFry 8-10 minutes until golden brown and the center is set. Transfer to a wire rack to cool completely. Serve.

Prosciutto & Mozzarella Bruschetta

Prep + Cook Time: 7 minutes 2 Servings

Ingredients

- ½ cup tomatoes, finely chopped

- 3 oz mozzarella cheese, grated

- 3 prosciutto slices, chopped

- 1 tbsp olive oil

- 1 tsp dried basil

- 6 small French bread slices

Directions

Preheat air fryer to 350 F. Add in the bread slices and toast for 3 minutes on AirFry mode. Remove and top the bread with tomatoes, prosciutto, and mozzarella cheese. Sprinkle basil all over and drizzle with olive oil. Return to the fryer and cook for 1 more minute, just to heat through. Serve warm.

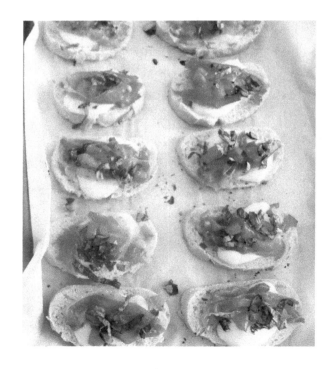

Mushroom & Chicken Mini Pizzas

Prep + Cook Time: 15 minutes 1 Serving

Ingredients

- ½ cup chicken meat, thinly chopped

- ¼ cup tomato-basil sauce

- 1 cup button mushrooms, sliced

- 1 tsp Parmesan cheese, grated

- 1 tsp black pepper

- ½ tsp garlic powder

Directions

Preheat air fryer to 400 F. Line a baking dish with parchment paper. In a bowl, combine chicken with garlic and pepper. Place spoonfuls of the chicken into the dish and flatten into rounds. AirFryfor 8-10 minutes, remove, turn, and top with tomato-basil sauce, mushrooms, and Parmesan cheese. Slide in the fryer and continue cooking for 5-6 minutes more until golden. Serve.

Soppressata Pizza

Prep + Cook Time: 15 minutes 2 Servings

Ingredients

- 1 pizza crust

- ½ tsp dried oregano

- ½ cup passata

- ½ cup mozzarella cheese, shredded

- 4 oz soppressata, chopped

- 4 basil leaves

Directions

Preheat air fryer to 370 F. Spread the passata over the pizza crust, sprinkle with oregano, mozzarella cheese, and finish with soppressata. Bake in the fryer for 10 minutes. Top with basil leaves to serve.

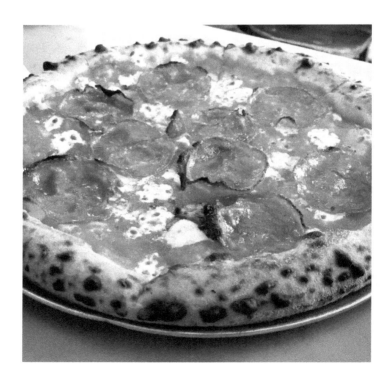

Sausage Frittata with Parmesan

Prep + Cook Time: 15 minutes 2 Servings

Ingredients

- 1 sausage, chopped

- Salt and black pepper to taste

- 1 tbsp parsley, chopped

- 4 eggs

- 1 tbsp olive oil

- 4 cherry tomatoes, halved

- 2 tbsp Parmesan cheese, shredded

Directions

Preheat air fryer to 360 F. Place tomatoes and sausages in the air fryer's basket and cook for 5 minutes. Remove them to a bowl and mix in eggs, salt, parsley, Parmesan cheese, olive oil, and black pepper. Add the mixture to a greased baking pan and fit in the fryer. Bake for 8 minutes. Serve hot.

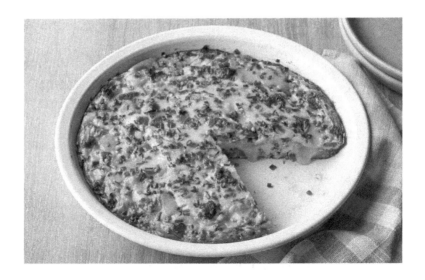

Crustless Broccoli & Mushroom Quiche

Prep + Cook Time: 25 minutes 4 Servings

Ingredients

- 4 eggs, beaten

- 1 cup mushrooms, sliced

- 1 cup broccoli florets, steamed

- ½ cup cheddar cheese, shredded

- ½ cup mozzarella cheese, shredded

- 2 tbsp olive oil

- ¼ tsp ground allspice

- Salt and black pepper to tast

Directions

Preheat air fryer to 360 F. Warm the olive oil in a pan over medium heat. Sauté the mushrooms for 3-4 minutes or until soft. Stir the broccoli for 1 minute; set aside. Put the eggs, cheddar cheese, mozzarella cheese, allspice, salt, and pepper in a medium bowl and whisk well. Pour the mushroom/broccoli concoction into the egg mixture and gently fold it in. Transfer the batter to a greased baking pan. Air fry for 5 minutes, then stir the mixture and air fry until the eggs are done, about 3-5 more minutes. Cut into wedges and serve.

Zucchini Muffins

Prep + Cook Time: 25 minutes 4 Servings

Ingredients

- 1 ½ cups flour

- 1 tsp cinnamon

- 3 eggs

- 2 tsp baking powder

- ½ tsp sugar

- 1 cup milk

- 2 tbsp butter, melted

- 1 tbsp yogurt

- 1 zucchini, shredded A pinch of salt

- 2 tbsp cream cheese

Directions

Preheat air fryer to 350 F. In a bowl, whisk the eggs with sugar, salt, cinnamon, cream cheese, flour, and baking powder. In another bowl, combine the remaining ingredients, except for the zucchini. Gently combine the dry and liquid mixtures. Stir in zucchini. Grease the muffin tins with cooking spray and pour the batter inside them. Place in the air fryer and cook for 18 minutes. Serve warm or chilled.

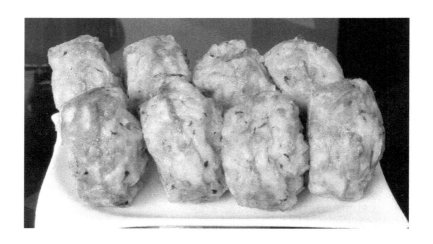

Banana & Hazelnut Muffins

Prep + Cook Time: 30 minutes 6 Servings

Ingredients

- ¼ cup butter, melted

- ¼ cup honey

- 1 egg, lightly beaten

- 2 ripe bananas, mashed

- ½ tsp vanilla extract

- 1 cup flour

- ½ tsp baking powder

- ½ tsp ground cinnamon

- ¼ cup hazelnuts, chopped

- ¼ cup dark chocolate chips

Directions

Spray a muffin tin that fits in your air fryer with cooking spray. In a bowl, whisk butter, honey, eggs, bananas, and vanilla until well combined. Sift in flour, baking powder, and cinnamon without overmixing. Stir in the hazelnuts and chocolate. Pour the batter into the muffin holes and fit in the air fryer. Cook for 20 minutes at 350 F on Bake, checking them around the 15-minute mark. Serve chilled.

Breakfast Banana Bread

Prep + Cook Time: 30 minutes 2 Servings

Ingredients

- 1 cup flour

- ¼ tsp baking soda

- 1 tsp baking powder

- 1/3 cup sugar

- 2 mashed bananas

- ¼ cup vegetable oil

- 1 egg, beaten

- 1 tsp vanilla extract

- ¾ cup chopped walnuts

- ¼ tsp salt

- 2 tbsp peanut butter, softened

- 2 tbsp sour cream

Directions

Preheat air fryer to 350 F. Sift the flour into a large bowl and add salt, baking powder, and baking soda; stir to combine. In another bowl, combine the bananas, vegetable oil, egg, peanut butter, vanilla, sugar, and sour cream; stir. Mix both mixtures and fold in the chopped walnuts. Pour the batter into a greased baking dish and fit in the fryer. Bake for 20-25 minutes until nice and golden. Serve chilled.

Sweet Bread Pudding with Raisins

Prep + Cook Time: 45 minutes 4 Servings

Ingredients

- 8 bread slices, cubed

- ½ cup buttermilk

- ¼ cup honey

- 1 cup milk

- 2 eggs

- ½ tsp vanilla extract

- 2 tbsp butter, softened

- ¼ cup sugar

- 4 tbsp raisins

- 2 tbsp chopped hazelnuts

- Ground cinnamon for garnish

Directions

Preheat air fryer to 350 F. Beat the eggs with buttermilk, honey, milk, vanilla, sugar, and butter in a bowl. Stir in raisins and hazelnuts, then add in the bread cubes to soak, about 10 minutes. Transfer to a greased tin and Bake the pudding in fryer for 25 minutes. Dust with ground cinnamon and serve.

Cherry & Almond Scones

Prep + Cook Time: 25 minutes 4 Servings

Ingredients

- 2 cups flour + some more

- 1/3 cup sugar

- 2 tsp baking powder

- ½ cup sliced almonds

- ¾ cup chopped cherries, dried

- ¼ cup cold butter, cut into cubes

- ½ cup milk 1 egg 1 tsp vanilla extract

Directions

Line the air fryer basket with baking paper. Mix together flour, sugar, baking powder, sliced almonds, and dried cherries in a bowl. Rub the butter into the dry ingredients with hands to form a sandy, crumbly texture. Whisk together egg, milk, and vanilla extract. Pour into the dry ingredients and stir to combine. Sprinkle a working board with flour, lay the dough onto the board, and give it a few kneads. Shape into a rectangle and cut into 9 squares. Arrange the squares in the air fryer's basket and cook for 14 minutes at 390 F. Work in batches if needed. Serve immediately.

Toasted Herb & Garlic Bagel

Prep + Cook Time: 10 minutes 1 Serving

Ingredients

- 1 tbsp butter, softened

- ¼ tsp dried basil

- ¼ tsp dried parsley

- ¼ tsp garlic powder

- 1 tbsp Parmesan cheese, grated

- Salt and black pepper to taste

- 1 bagel, halved

Directions

Preheat air fryer to 370 degrees. Place the bagel halves in the fryer and toast for 3 minutes on AirFry mode. Mix butter, Parmesan cheese, garlic, basil, and parsley in a bowl. Season with salt and pepper. Spread the mixture onto the toasted bagel and return to the fryer to AirFry for 3 more minutes. Serve.

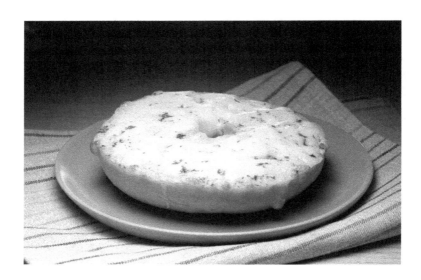

Spanish Chorizo Frittata

Prep + Cook Time: 20 minutes 2 Servings

Ingredients

- 4 eggs

- 1 large potato, boiled and cubed

- ½ cup sweet corn

- ½ cup feta cheese, crumbled

- 1 tbsp parsley, chopped

- 1 chorizo sausage, sliced

- 2 tbsp olive oil

- Salt and black pepper to taste

Directions

Preheat air fryer to 330 F. Heat olive oil in a skillet over medium heat and cook the chorizo until slightly browned, about 4 minutes; set aside. In a bowl, beat the eggs with salt and black pepper. Stir in all of the remaining ingredients, except for the parsley. Grease a baking pan that fits your air fryer with the chorizo fat and pour in the egg mixture. Insert into the air fryer and Bake for 8-10 minutes until golden. Serve topped with parsley. Enjoy!

Easy Breakfast Potatoes

Prep + Cook Time: 35 minutes 6 Servings

Ingredients

- 4 large potatoes, cubed

- 2 bell peppers, cut into

- 1-inch chunks

- ½ onion, diced

- 2 tsp olive oil

- 1 garlic clove, minced

- ½ tsp dried thyme

- ½ tsp cayenne pepper Salt to taste

Directions Preheat air fryer to 390 F. Place the potato cubes in a bowl and sprinkle with garlic, cayenne pepper, and salt. Drizzle with some olive oil and toss to coat. Arrange the potatoes on an even layer on the greased air fryer basket. Air Fry for 10 minutes, shaking the basket once during the cooking time. In the meantime, add the remaining olive oil, garlic, thyme, and salt in a mixing bowl. Add in the bell peppers and onion and mix well. Pour the veggies over the potatoes and continue cooking in the air fryer for 5 minutes. At the 5-minute mark, shake the basket and cook for 5 minutes. Serve warm.

Air Fried Shirred Eggs

Prep + Cook Time: 20 minutes 2 Servings

Ingredients

- 2 tsp butter

- 4 eggs

- 2 tbsp heavy cream

- 4 slices ham

- 3 tbsp Parmesan cheese, grated

- ¼ tsp paprika

- Salt and black pepper to taste

- 2 tsp chopped chives

Directions

Preheat air fryer to 320 F. Arrange the ham slices on the bottom of a greased pie pan to cover it completely. Whisk one egg along with the heavy cream, salt, and pepper in a small bowl. Pour the mixture over the ham slices. Crack the other eggs on top and sprinkle with Parmesan cheese. AirFry for 14 minutes. Garnish with paprika and fresh chives and serve.

Pancake The German Way

Prep + Cook Time: 30 minutes 4 Servings

Ingredients

- 3 eggs, beaten

- 2 tbsp butter, melted

- 1 cup flour 2 tbsp sugar, powdered

- ½ cup milk

- 1 cup fresh strawberries, sliced

Directions

Preheat air fryer to 330 F. In a bowl, mix flour, milk, and eggs until fully incorporated. Grease a baking pan that fits in your air fryer with the butter and pour in the mixture. Place the pan in the air fryer's basket and AirFry for 12-16 minutes until the pancake is fluffy and golden brown. Drizzle powdered sugar and arrange sliced strawberries on top to serve.

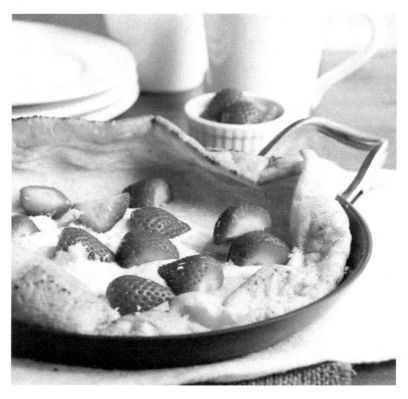

Masala Omelet the Indian Way

Prep + Cook Time: 15 minutes 1 Serving

Ingredients

- 1 garlic clove, crushed

- 2 green onions

- ½ chili powder

- ½ tsp garam masala

- 2 eggs

- 1 tbsp olive oil

- 1 tbsp fresh cilantro, chopped

- Salt and black pepper to taste

Directions

Warm the olive oil in a skillet over medium. Add and sauté the spring onions and garlic for 2 minutes until softened. Sprinkle with chili powder, garam masala, salt, and pepper. Set aside. Preheat air fryer to 340 F. In a bowl, mix the eggs with salt and black pepper. Add in the masala mixture and stir well. Transfer to a greased baking that fits into your air fryer. Bake in the fryer for 8 minutes until golden, flipping once. Scatter your omelet with cilantro and serve immediately.

Three Meat Cheesy Omelet

Prep + Cook Time: 20 minutes 2 Servings

Ingredients

- 1 beef sausage, chopped

- 4 slices prosciutto, chopped

- 3 oz salami, chopped

- 1 cup mozzarella cheese, grated

- 4 eggs

- 1 green onion, chopped

- 1 tbsp ketchup

- 1 tsp fresh parsley, chopped

Directions

Preheat air fryer to 350 F. Whisk the eggs with ketchup in a bowl. Stir in green onion, mozzarella, salami, and prosciutto. AirFry the sausage in a greased baking tray in the fryer for 2 minutes. Slide-out and pour the egg mixture on top. Cook for another 8 minutes until golden. Serve sliced with parsley.

Orange Creamy Cupcakes

Prep + Cook Time: 25 minutes 4 Servings

Ingredients

Lemon Frosting:

- 1 cup plain yogurt

- 2 tbsp sugar

- 1 orange, juiced

- 1 tbsp orange zest

- 7 oz cream cheese

Cake:

- 2 lemons, seeded and quartered

- ½ cup flour + extra for basing

- ¼ tsp salt

- 2 tbsp sugar

- 1 tsp baking powder

- 1 tsp vanilla extract

- 2 eggs

- ½ cup butter, softened

- 2 tbsp milk

Directions

In a bowl, add yogurt and cream cheese and mix until smooth. Add in orange juice and zest and whisk well. Gradually add the sugar and stir until smooth. Make sure the frost is not runny. Set aside. Place the lemon quarters in a food processor and process until pureed. Add in the flour, baking powder, softened butter, milk, eggs, vanilla extract, sugar, and salt. Process again until smooth. Preheat air fryer to 360 F. Flour the bottom of 4 cupcake cases and spoon the batter into the cases, ¾ way up. Place them in the air fryer and bake for 12 minutes or until the inserted toothpick comes out clean. Once ready, remove and let cool. Design the cupcakes with the frosting and serve.

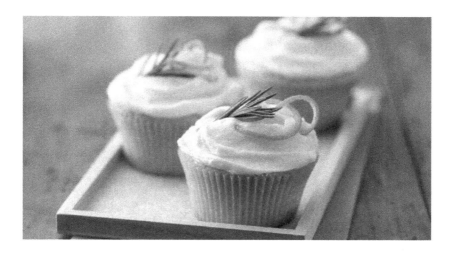

Avocado Tempura

Prep + Cook Time: 10 minutes 4 Servings

Ingredients

- ½ cup breadcrumbs

- ½ tsp salt

- 1 avocado, pitted, peeled, and sliced

- ½ cup liquid from beans

Directions

Preheat air fryer to 360 F. In a bowl, add the crumbs and salt and mix to combine. Sprinkle the avocado with the beans' liquid and then coat in the crumbs. Arrange the slices in one layer inside the fryer and AirFry for 8-10 minutes, shaking once or twice. Serve warm

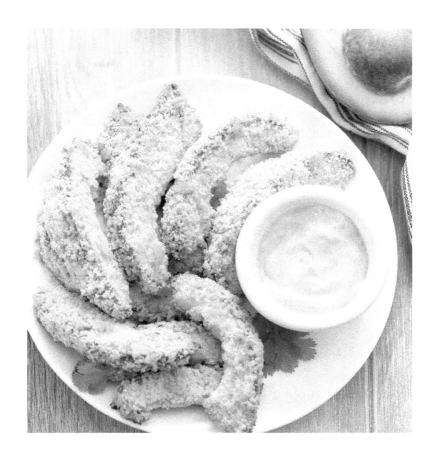

Blueberry Oat Bars

Prep + Cook Time: 20 minutes 12 bars

Ingredients

- 2 cups rolled oats

- ¼ cup ground almonds

- ¼ cup sugar

- 1 tsp baking powder

- ½ tsp ground cinnamon

- 2 eggs, lightly beaten

- ½ cup canola oil

- ½ cup milk

- 1 tsp vanilla extract

- 2 cups blueberries

Directions

Spray a baking pan that fits in your air fryer with cooking spray. In a bowl, add oats, almonds, sugar, baking powder, and cinnamon and stir well. In another bowl, whisk eggs, canola oil, milk, and vanilla. Stir the wet ingredients gently into the oat mixture. Fold in the blueberries. Pour the mixture into the pan and place it in the fryer. Cook for 10 minutes at 350 F. Let it cool on a wire rack. Cut into 12 bars.

Crispy Croutons

Prep + Cook Time: 20 minutes 4 Servings

Ingredients

- 2 cups bread cubes

- 2 tbsp butter, melted

- 1 tsp dried parsley

- Garlic salt and black pepper to taste

Directions

Mix the cubed bread with butter, parsley, garlic salt, and black pepper until well coated. Place in the fryer's basket and AirFry for 6-8 minutes at 380 F, shaking once until golden brown. Use in soups.

Roasted Asparagus with Serrano Ham

Prep + Cook Time: 15 minutes 4 Servings

Ingredients

- 12 spears asparagus, trimmed

- 12 Serrano ham slices

- ¼ cup Parmesan cheese, grated

- Salt and black pepper to taste

Directions

Preheat air fryer to 350 F. Season asparagus with salt and black pepper. Wrap each ham slice around each asparagus spear from one end to the other end to cover completely.

Arrange them on the greased air fryer basket and AirFry for 10 minutes, shaking once or twice throughout cooking. When ready, scatter with Parmesan cheese and serve immediately.

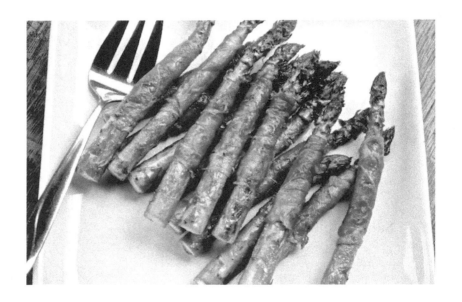

Very Berry Breakfast Puffs

Prep + Cook Time: 20 minutes 4 Servings

Ingredients

- 1 puff pastry sheet

- 1 tbsp strawberries, mashed

- 1 tbsp raspberries, mashed

- ¼ tsp vanilla extract

- 1 cup cream cheese

- 1 tbsp honey

Directions

Preheat air fryer to 375 F. Roll the puff pastry out on a lightly floured surface into a 1-inch thick rectangle. Cut into 4 squares. Spread the cream cheese evenly on them. In a bowl, combine the berries, honey, and vanilla. Spoon the mixture onto the pastry squares. Fold in the sides over the filling. Pinch the ends to form a puff. Place the puffs on a lined with waxed paper baking dish. Bake in the air fryer for 15 minutes until the pastry is puffed and golden all over. Let it cool for 10 mins before serving.

THANK YOU

Thank you for choosing *Low Fat Air Fryer Breakfast Meal Prep* for improving your cooking skills! I hope you enjoyed making the recipes as much as tasting them! If you're interested in learning new recipes and new meals to cook, go and check out the other books of the series.

CPSIA information can be obtained
at www.ICGtesting.com
Printed in the USA
BVHW090024140521
607263BV00002B/136